A is for Anger
How to Cope:
The Medical Librarian's
Annotated Guide

By William Jiang, MLS

This is a work of nonfiction.

None of the passages in this book should be understood or construed as a recommendation or condemnation of any particular drug, medication, or treatment for anger or any other mental illness. Further, the author is a medical librarian, not a doctor, so consult your doctor with any medical questions that may arise.

Copyright (c) 2016 by William Jiang

All rights reserved. Printed in the United States of America. No part of this book may be reproduced in any manner whatsoever without written pernlission except in the case of brief quotations embodied in critical articles and reviews for information, address kd3qc@yahoo.com

ISBN-13: 978-1541003316
ISBN-10: 1541003314

Jiang, William, 1972-
A is for Anger: How to Cope- The Medical Librarian's Annotated Guide

William Jiang
170 p.
l. Jiang, William, 1972-.2. Anger

For my Amor, eres todas mis razones!
"Vivir es Amar."
"To live is to love"

A is for Anger: How to Cope-
The Medical Librarian's Annotated Guide
William Jiang, MLS

Anger. It is a common emotion at all ages which can run the gambit from feeling a little peeved to homicidal rage. Plato said, There are two things a person should never be angry at, what they can help, and what they cannot. Aristotle said, Anybody can become angry - that is easy, but to be angry with the right person and to the right degree and at the right time and for the right purpose, and in the right way - that is not within everybody's power and is not easy. Indeed, to feel anger is a healthy emotion. If one represses anger habitually, it is as a kettle that is being heated without allowing steam to escape. As the teapot would, the person will eventually explode with anger.

However, anger can become a problem when it is unwarranted, exaggerated, or extreme. Anger is primarily a health problem that not only affects the people around the person with anger, but also they are damaging themselves, raising the risk of things like a heart attack. Also, it can damage one's social circle by putting one in less fun environments like prison or psychiatric settings. Indeed, people with intermittent explosive disorder and impulsive aggression often possess a dysfunctional connection between regions of the brain that are associated with sensory input, language processing and social interaction.

Life can make one angry, as can circumstances, especially when life is viewed as "unfair". Medical conditions can aggravate this feeling of unfairness such as anxiety, bipolar, depression, schizophrenia, drug or alcohol abuse, as well as eating disorders, You may wish to check out my other book **Guide to Natural Mental Health: Anxiety, Bipolar, Depression, Schizophrenia, and Digital Addiction: Nutrition, and Complementary Therapies** to treat underlying issues that may be making you angry.

All that being said, what can one do to lessen and prevent anger? The following annotated bibliography contains seeds of wisdom about how one can mitigate and help people who may be struggling with anger issues: from increasing potassium in the diet to reducing sodium, from natural diet and lifestyle interventions, to helpful medications such as the antidepressant SSRIs and certain antipsychotics. Librarians use annotated bibliographies in an attempts to survey the literature in a discipline, and present the information in notes which are easily understood, cutting through the medical jargon. The present annotated bibliography about anger presents the insights and work of over eighty medical researchers around the globe.

I wish you hope and healing.

In Health
William Jiang, MLS

TABLE OF CONTENTS

- Multivitamin, Multi-Mineral Supplements and Anger
- Salt and Anger
- Calorie Restriction and Anger
- Caffeine, Smoking, and Drinking and Anger
- Anger and Heart Attacks
- The Circadian Rhythm and Anger
- Temperature and Anger
- Apps and Anger
- CBT and Anger Management
- Nature and Anger
- Yoga and Meditation and Anger
- Zinc and Anger
- Vitamin D and Anger
- Iron and Anger

- Dairy and Anger
- Leucine May Fight Anger
- Controlling Anger with Medication
- Aspirin, Antidepressants, and Anger
- Risperidone and Anger

Multivitamin, Multi-Mineral Supplements and Anger

Take a multivitamin if you deal with anger. It is the easiest and first intervention everybody should take to mitigate anger.

Biomed Environ Sci. 2013 Jul;26(7):599-604. doi: 10.3967/0895-3988.2013.07.012.
Effects of a multivitamin/multimineral supplement on young males with physical overtraining: a placebo-controlled, randomized, double-blinded cross-over trial.
Li X1, Huang WX, Lu JM, Yang G, Ma FL, Lan YT, Meng JH, Dou JT.
Author information
Abstract
OBJECTIVE:
To investigate the effects of vitamin-mineral supplement on young males with physical overtraining.
METHODS:
Two hundred and forty male Chinese field artillery personnel who undertook large scale and endurance military training and were on ordinary Chinese diet were randomized to receive a multivitamin/multimineral supplement or a placebo for 1 week. After a 1-week wash-out period, a cross-over with 1 week course of a placebo or multivitamin/multimineral

supplement was conducted. Blood and urine samples were analyzed for adrenal, gonadal and thyroid hormones. In addition, cellular immune parameters (CD3+, CD3+CD4+, CD3+CD8+, CD4/CD8, CD3-CD56+, CD3-CD19+) were examined and psychological tests were performed before and after the training program and nutrition intervention.

RESULTS:

After a large scale and endurance military training, the participants showed significantly increased thyroid function, decreased adrenal cortex, testosterone and immunological function, and significantly increased somatization, anger and tension. Compared to placebo, multivitamin/ multimineral intervention showed significant effects on functional recovery of the pituitary - adrenal axis, pituitary-gonadal axis, pituitary- thyroid axis and immune system as well as psychological parameters.

CONCLUSION:

High-intensity military operations have significant impacts on the psychology, physical ability and neuroendocrine-immune system in young males. **Appropriate supplementation of multivitamin/multimineral can facilitate the recovery of the psychology, physical ability and neuroendocrine-immune system in young males who take ordinary Chinese diet.**

Copyright © 2013 The Editorial Board of Biomedi-

cal and Environmental Sciences. Published by China CDC. All rights reserved.
KEYWORDS:
Diet supplement; Intervention; Overtraining; Randomized; Vitamins
PMID: 23895706 DOI: 10.3967/0895-3988.2013.07.012
[PubMed - indexed for MEDLINE] Free full text

Salt and Anger

A low-sodium, high-potassium diet (LNAHK) can help to control anger. Decrease your table salt consumption and increase the potassium in your diet to benefit.

Top 7 Potassium Rich Foods List

1. *Avocado. 1 whole: 1068 mg (30% DV)*
2. *Spinach. 1 cup: 839mg (24% DV)*
3. *Sweet potato. 1 medium: 952 mg (27% DV)*

4. *Coconut Water. 1 cup 600 mg (17% DV)*
5. *Kefir or Yogurt. 1 cup: 579 mg (15% DV)*
6. *White Beans. ½ cup: 502 mg (15% DV)*
7. *Banana. 1 large: 422 mg (12% DV)*

Br J Nutr. 2008 Nov;100(5):1038-45. doi: 10.1017/S0007114508959201. Epub 2008 May 9.
Dietary electrolytes are related to mood.
Torres SJ1, Nowson CA, Worsley A.
Author information
Abstract
Dietary therapies are routinely recommended to reduce disease risk; however, there is concern they may adversely affect mood. We compared the effect on mood of a low-sodium, high-potassium diet (LNAHK) and a high-calcium diet (HC) with a moderate-sodium, high-potassium, high-calcium Dietary Approaches to Stop Hypertension (DASH)-type diet (OD). We also assessed the relationship between dietary electrolytes and cortisol, a stress hormone and marker of hypothalamic-pituitary-adrenal (HPA) axis activity. In a crossover design, subjects were randomized to two diets for 4 weeks, the OD and either LNAHK or HC, each preceded by a 2-week control diet (CD). Dietary compliance was assessed by 24 h urine collections. Mood was measured weekly by the Profile of Mood States

(POMS). Saliva samples were collected to measure cortisol. The change in mood between the preceding CD and the test diet (LNAHK or HC) was compared with the change between the CD and OD. Of the thirty-eight women and fifty-six men (mean age 56.3 (sem 9.8) years) that completed the OD, forty-three completed the LNAHK and forty-eight the HC. **There was a greater improvement in depression, tension, vigour and the POMS global score for the LNAHK diet compared to OD ($P < 0.05$).** Higher cortisol levels were weakly associated with greater vigour, lower fatigue, and higher levels of urinary potassium and magnesium (r 0.1-0.2, $P < 0.05$ for all). In conclusion, a LNAHK diet appeared to have a positive effect on overall mood.

PMID: 18466657 DOI: 10.1017/S0007114508959201

[PubMed - indexed for MEDLINE]

Caffeine, Smoking, and Drinking and Anger

The following two articles indicate that If one has anger issues, it is best to avoid smoking and drinking, period, especially starting in adolescence. Beware the person who is inebriated who turns their anger onto themselves or others. Although difficult, it is best to avoid caffeine as well.

Nicotine Tob Res. 2014 Aug;16(8):1085-93. doi: 10.1093/ntr/ntu033. Epub 2014 Apr 1.
Hostility and cigarette use: a comparison between smokers and nonsmokers in a matched sample of adolescents.
Bernstein MH1, Colby SM2, Bidwell LC2, Kahler CW3, Leventhal AM4.
Author information
Abstract
INTRODUCTION:
We examined the association between hostility-a personality trait reflective of negativity and cynicism toward others-and smoking in adolescents by measuring (a) several subcomponents of hostility, and (b) facial emotion processing ability, which has been previously linked to hostility.
METHODS:
Participants (N = 241 aged 14-19) were 95 smokers and 95 demographically matched nonsmokers as well

as 51 nonmatched smokers. All participants completed the Cook-Medley (C-M) hostility scale, which provides a general hostility score and 3 component scores (cynicism, hypersensitivity, and aggressive responding), and a facial emotion processing task. This task, designed to assess emotion recognition, requires quickly identifying the emotion of faces that gradually morph from neutral to high-intensity happy, angry, or fearful.

RESULTS:

Independent sample t tests indicated that matched smokers scored significantly higher in cynicism and aggressive responding than nonsmokers. Among smokers, age of smoking onset was negatively correlated with general hostility and aggressive responding. All hostility scales were positively correlated with the intensity needed to recognize happy faces. Counterintuitively, smokers required a greater intensity to recognize angry faces than nonsmokers. No other relations between hostility/smoking status and facial emotion processing were observed.

CONCLUSIONS:

Aspects of hostility, particularly aggressive responding, may be a risk factor for early onset smoking. Although hostile participants exhibited a deficiency in their ability to recognize happiness in facial pictures, these results did not translate to differences in smoking status. This study elucidates some of the complex interrelations between hostility, emotion processing, and adolescent smoking, which may have implications for teen smoking prevention.

© The Author 2014. Published by Oxford University Press on behalf of the Society for Research on Nicotine and Tobacco. All rights reserved. For permissions, please e-mail: journals.permissions@oup.com.
PMID: 24692670 PMCID: PMC4155423 DOI: 10.1093/ntr/ntu033

Subst Use Misuse. 2015 Jan;50(2):257-67. doi: 10.3109/10826084.2014.977394. Epub 2014 Nov 20.
A gender-specific analysis of adolescent dietary caffeine, alcohol consumption, anger, and violent behavior.
James JE1, Kristjansson AL, Sigfusdottir ID.
Author information
Abstract
Self-reported dietary caffeine and alcohol consumption were examined in relation to anger and violent behavior in Icelandic tenth-graders. Structural equation modeling (SEM) was used to investigate direct and indirect effects of measured and latent variables in the population sample of 3,670, controlling for parental financial standing, family structure, ADHD, and peer delinquency. Gender differences were observed that have not been reported previously, espe-

cially in relation to anger as a possible mediator of violent behavior against a background of caffeine and alcohol consumption. **Study findings suggest the need to take account of caffeine consumption in relation to adolescent anger and violence.**
KEYWORDS:
adolescence; adolescents; alcohol; anger; caffeine; gender differences; violence

Anger and Heart Attacks

Anger can cause heart attacks.

Circulation. 1991 Apr;83(4 Suppl):II81-9.
Autonomic nervous system and coronary blood flow changes related to emotional activation and sleep.
Verrier RL1, Dickerson LW.
Author information

Abstract

Experimental models have been developed to investigate the influences of anger, fear, and sleep on coronary blood flow. **Studies of anger in dogs with coronary stenosis indicate that the postarousal phase is particularly conducive to myocardial ischemia.** Specifically, a delayed coronary vasoconstrictor response has been observed within 1-3 minutes after cessation of behavioral arousal. The response is prevented by bilateral stellectomy and can be elicited in anesthetized animals by electrical stimulation of the right or left stellate ganglion. The latter effect is averted by alpha-adrenergic blockade with prazosin. Although the basis for the protracted nature of the delayed vasoconstriction remains to be clarified, the current hypothesis is that the phenomenon results from a time-dependent imbalance between the vasoconstrictor effects of adrenergic input and the vasodilator influences of coronary pressure and/or cardiac metabolic activity. A behavioral model emulating the fear state has also been developed. When dogs that fail to exhibit anger are placed in a food-access confrontation protocol, the animals demonstrate a fearlike state evidenced by a cowering posture and somatic tremor. There is a distinct plasma catecholamine profile that is characterized by a predominant increase in epinephrine compared with norepinephrine. This is in contrast to the pattern observed

during anger, in which a prevalent increase in norepinephrine is observed. Fear results in significant increases in heart rate, arterial blood pressure, and coronary arterial flow. Sleep is also associated with substantial alterations in coronary hemodynamic function.(ABSTRACT TRUNCATED AT 250 WORDS)
PMID: 2009632
[PubMed - indexed for MEDLINE]

The Circadian Rhythm and Anger

Disrupted sleep can cause anger, sporadically. Chronically tired people can develop chronic anger and psychiatric issues. Healthy sleep is important for everybody.

Med Hypotheses. 2011 Oct;77(4):692-5. doi: 10.1016/j.mehy.2011.07.019. Epub 2011 Aug 9.
Severe mood dysregulation: in the "light" of circa-

dian functioning.

Heiler S1, Legenbauer T, Bogen T, Jensch T, Holtmann M.

Author information

Abstract

Severe affective and behavioral dysregulation, labeled as severe mood dysregulation (SMD), is a widely spread phenomenon among adolescent psychiatric patients. This phenotype constitutes severe impairment across multiple settings, including various symptoms, such as non-episodic anger, mood instability, and hyperarousal. Moreover, SMD patients often show depression and reduced need for sleep. Despite a lifetime prevalence of 3.3%, systematic research is still scarce, and treatments that have been established do not account for the range of symptoms present in SMD. **Considering the circadian dysfunctions, two hormones, melatonin and cortisol, are essential. When these hormones are dysregulated, the circadian rhythm gets out of synchrony. Since evidence is emerging showing that the worse the sleep-wake cycle is entrained, the worse the psychiatric symptoms are depicted, the importance of proper circadian functioning becomes clear.** Chronotherapy as the controlled exposure to environmental stimuli (e.g. light) acting on biological rhythms has shown therapeutic effects. In both seasonal and major depression chronotherapy has been implemented, decreasing depressive symptoms and stabilizing circadian rhythms. Preliminary evidence from SMD related disorders, namely attention-deficit/hyperactivity disorder and pediatric bipolar depression, indicates that morning light therapy elicits positive influences on other symptoms as well. Hence, light therapy might not only be effective for depressive symptoms and circadian rhythms, but might also be beneficial for symptoms including inattention and irritability. We hypothesize that light therapy might be a helpful adjunctive treatment enhancing affective and circadian functioning, and eliciting positive influences on behavior. Physiologically, changes of both cortisol levels and melatonin production are expected.

Copyright © 2011 Elsevier Ltd. All rights reserved.
PMID: 21831530 DOI: 10.1016/j.mehy.2011.07.019

Temperature and Anger

When people are feeling too hot, they may get angry more often.

Environ Res. 2016 Nov;151:124-129. doi: 10.1016/j.envres.2016.06.045. Epub 2016 Jul 29.
Increasing ambient temperature reduces emotional well-being.
Noelke C1, McGovern M2, Corsi DJ3, Jimenez MP4, Stern A5, Wing IS5, Berkman L6.
Author information
Abstract
This study examines the impact of ambient temperature on emotional well-being in the U.S. population aged 18+. The U.S. is an interesting test case because of its resources, technology and variation in climate across different areas, which also allows us to examine whether adaptation to different climates could weaken or even eliminate the impact of heat on well-being. Using survey responses from 1.9 million Americans over the period from 2008 to 2013, we estimate the effect of temperature on well-being from exogenous day-to-day temperature variation within respondents' area of residence and test whether this effect varies across areas with different climates. We find that increasing temperatures significantly reduce well-being. **Compared to average daily tempera-**

tures in the 50-60°F (10-16°C) range, temperatures above 70°F (21°C) reduce positive emotions (e.g. joy, happiness), increase negative emotions (e.g. stress, anger), and increase fatigue (feeling tired, low energy). These effects are particularly strong among less educated and older Americans. However, there is no consistent evidence that heat effects on well-being differ across areas with mild and hot summers, suggesting limited variation in heat adaptation.

Copyright © 2016 Elsevier Inc. All rights reserved.

KEYWORDS:

Climate impacts; Heat exposure; Mental health; Social inequality; Subjective well-being

Apps and Anger

There's an app for that. There are apps that can help with anger management.

Mil Med. 2016 Sep;181(9):990-5. doi: 10.7205/MILMED-D-15-00293.
Using a Mobile Application in the Management of Anger Problems Among Veterans: A Pilot Study.
Morland LA1, Niehaus J2, Taft C3, Marx BP3, Menez U4, Mackintosh MA1.
Author information
Abstract
OBJECTIVE:
This feasibility pilot study evaluated the usability of a mobile application (app), Remote Exercises for Learning Anger and Excitation Management (RELAX), as an adjunct to an anger management treatment delivered to Veterans.
METHODS:
Four Veterans completed pre- and post-treatment measures of anger, post-traumatic stress disorder, depression, interpersonal functioning, and app use.
RESULTS:
Descriptive results of clinical outcomes are provided. Qualitative data included Veterans' and therapists' feedback regarding the acceptability of the technology, satisfaction with the RELAX app, homework

facilitation, and suggestions for improvement. Large reductions in anger, post-traumatic stress disorder and depression symptoms, and improvements in social functioning were evidenced post-treatment. Veterans reported that the RELAX app was helpful and appreciated its functionality.
CONCLUSIONS:
Our findings support using an app as an adjunct to traditional anger management.
Reprint & Copyright © 2016 Association of Military Surgeons of the U.S.
PMID: 27612342 DOI: 10.7205/MILMED-D-15-00293

CBT and Anger Management

Psychologists have developed great tools for anger management. Anger management techniques in combination with lifestyle interventions can make anger better. CBT or Cognitive Behavioral Therapy is one of the gold standard techniques of psychology.

Behav Cogn Psychother. 2016 Sep 15:1-15. [Epub ahead of print]
CBT in a Caribbean Context: A Controlled Trial of Anger Management in Trinidadian Prisons.
Hutchinson G1, Willner P2, Rose J3, Burke I4, Bastick T1.
Author information
Abstract
BACKGROUND:
Anger causes significant problems in offenders and to date few interventions have been described in the Caribbean region.
AIM:
To evaluate a package of CBT-based Anger Management Training provided to offenders in prison in Trinidad.
METHOD:
A controlled clinical trial with 85 participants who participated in a 12-week prison-based group anger management programme, of whom 57 (67%: 16 control, 41 intervention) provided pretrial and posttrial outcome data at Times 1 and 2.
RESULTS:
Intervention and control groups were not directly comparable so outcome was analysed using t-tests. **Reductions were noted for state and trait anger**

and anger expression, with an increase in coping skills for the intervention group. No changes were noted in the control group. The improvements seen on intervention were maintained at 4 month follow-up for a sub-group of participants for whom data were available. Several predictors of outcomes were identified.
KEYWORDS:
CBT; Caribbean; Trinidad; anger; controlled trial; prison
PMID: 27629438 DOI: 10.1017/S1352465816000266

Nature and Anger

When you are angry, instead of acting out on that anger, go for a walk in nature to clear your head or go chop wood until you are tired, there is evidence for this intervention.

Environ Sci Technol. 2011 Mar 1;45(5):1761-72. doi: 10.1021/es102947t. Epub 2011 Feb 3.

Does participating in physical activity in outdoor natural environments have a greater effect on physical and mental wellbeing than physical activity indoors? A systematic review.

Thompson Coon J1, Boddy K, Stein K, Whear R, Barton J, Depledge MH.

Author information

Abstract

Our objective was to compare the effects on mental and physical wellbeing, health related quality of life and long-term adherence to physical activity, of participation in physical activity in natural environments compared with physical activity indoors. We conducted a systematic review using the following data sources: Medline, Embase, Psychinfo, GreenFILE, SportDISCUS, The Cochrane Library, Science Citation Index Expanded, Social Sciences Citation Index, Arts and Humanities Citation Index, Conference Proceedings Citation Index--Science and BIOSIS from inception to June 2010. Internet searches of relevant Web sites, hand searches of relevant journals, and the reference lists of included papers and other review papers identified in the search were also searched for relevant information. Controlled trials (randomized and nonrandomized) were included. To be eligible trials had to compare the effects of outdoor exercise initiatives with those conducted indoors and report on at least one physical or mental wellbeing outcome in adults or children. Screening of articles for inclusion, data extraction, and quality appraisal were performed by one reviewer and checked by a second with discrepancies resolved by discussion with a third if necessary. Due to the heterogeneity of identified studies a narrative synthesis was performed. Eleven trials (833 adults) were included. Most participants (6 trials; 523 adults) were young students. Study entry criteria and methods were sparsely reported. All interventions consisted of a single episode of walking or running indoors with the same activity at a similar level conducted outdoors on a separate occasion. A total of 13 different outcome measures were used to evaluate the effects of exercise on mental wellbeing, and 4 outcome measures were used to assess attitude to exercise. Most trials (n = 9) showed some improvement in mental wellbeing on one or other of the outcome measures. **Compared with exercising indoors, exercising in natural environments was associated with greater feelings of revitalization and positive engagement, decreases in tension, confusion, anger, and depression, and increased energy.** However, the results suggested that feelings of calmness may be decreased following outdoor exercise. Participants reported greater enjoyment and satisfaction with outdoor activity and declared a greater intent to repeat the activity at a later date. None of the identified studies measured the effects of physical activity on physical wellbeing or the effect of natural environments on exercise adherence. The hypothesis that there are added beneficial effects to be gained from performing physical activity outdoors in natural environments is very appealing and has generated considerable interest. This review has shown some promising effects on self-reported mental wellbeing immediately following exercise in nature which are not seen following the same exercise indoors. However, the interpretation and extrapolation of these findings is hampered by the poor methodological quality of the available evidence and the heterogeneity of outcome measures employed. The review demonstrates the paucity of high quality evidence on which to base recommendations and reveals an undoubted need for further research in this area. Large, well designed, longer term trials in populations who might benefit most from the potential advantages of outdoor exercise are needed to fully elucidate the effects on mental and physical wellbeing. The influence of these effects on the sustainability of physical activity initiatives also awaits investigation.

Comment in

The benefits of being green. [Environ Sci Technol. 2012]

PMID: 21291246 DOI: 10.1021/es102947t
[PubMed - indexed for MEDLINE]

Yoga and Meditation and Anger

Physical and breathing yogic techniques as well as meditation can significantly help people with anger issues. Usually, best results start to occur after about eight weeks of regular practice, but benefits will accrue the longer yoga and meditation are practiced.

Int J Offender Ther Comp Criminol. 2016 Feb 22. pii: 0306624X16633667. [Epub ahead of print]
Mindfulness and Rehabilitation: Teaching Yoga and Meditation to Young Men in an Alternative to Incarceration Program.
Barrett CJ1.
Author information
Abstract
This study used participant/observation and open-ended interviews to understand how male partici-

pants (age 18-24 years) benefited from yoga and mindfulness training within an Alternative to Incarceration (ATI) program. Findings suggest that the male participants (age 18-24 years) benefited from the intervention through reductions in stress and improvements in emotion regulation. Several participants noted the importance of the development of an embodied practice for assisting them in managing anger and impulse control. The young men's narratives suggest that mindfulness-based interventions can contribute positively to rehabilitative outcomes within alternative to incarcerations settings, providing complementary benefit to existing ATI programs, especially for clients amenable to mindfulness training. With many jurisdictions expanding rehabilitation-focused interventions for young offenders, service providers should consider the potential positive contributions that mindfulness-based interventions can have for fostering desistance and reducing recidivism among justice system-involved populations.
© The Author(s) 2016.
KEYWORDS:
alternatives to incarceration; anger management; emotion regulation; mindfulness; rehabilitation; stress; youthful offenders
PMID: 26903231 DOI: 10.1177/0306624X16633667
[PubMed - as supplied by publisher]

Zinc and Anger

Make sure you get enough zinc in your diet, especially if you are male, and especially if you have anger issues. Do not supplement with too much zinc as it can be toxic.

Eur J Clin Nutr. 2010 Mar;64(3):331-3. doi: 10.1038/ejcn.2009.158. Epub 2010 Jan 20.
Effect of zinc supplementation on mood states in young women: a pilot study.
Sawada T1, Yokoi K.
Author information
Abstract
The relation of zinc (Zn) nutriture to brain development and function has been elucidated. The purpose of this study is to examine whether Zn supplementation improves mood states in young women. The study used a double-blind, randomized and placebo-controlled procedure. The major outcomes were psychological measures, somatic symptoms and serum Zn. Thirty women were placed randomly and in equal numbers into two groups, and they ingested one capsule containing multivitamins (MVs) or MV and 7 mg Zn daily for 10 weeks. Women who took MV and Zn showed a significant reduction in anger-hostility score ($P=0.009$) and depression-dejection score ($P=0.011$) in the Profile of Moods

State (POMS) and a significant increase in serum Zn concentration (P=0.008), whereas women who took only MV did not. **Our results suggest that Zn supplementation may be effective in reducing anger and depression.**
PMID: 20087376 DOI: 10.1038/ejcn.2009.158
[PubMed - indexed for MEDLINE]

Vitamin D and Anger

Make sure your vitamin D levels are normal if you are dealing with anger. Most people in developed nations would benefit from vitamin D supplementation.

J Diabetes Metab Disord. 2015 Jul 22;14:62. doi: 10.1186/s40200-015-0191-9. eCollection 2015.
The association of vitamin D deficiency with psychiatric distress and violence behaviors in Iranian adolescents: the CASPIAN-III study.
Ataie-Jafari A1, Qorbani M2, Heshmat R3, Ardalan G4, Motlagh ME5, Asayesh H6, Arzaghi SM7,

Tajadini MH8, Nejatinamini S3, Poursafa P4, Kelishadi R4.
Author information
Abstract
BACKGROUND:
Subtle effects of vitamin D deficiency on behavior have been suggested. We investigated the association of vitamin D status with mental health and violence behaviors in a sample of Iranian adolescents.
METHODS:
This nationwide study was conducted in 2009-2010 in 1095 Iranian school students with mean age 14.7 ± 2.6 years. Items were adapted from the Global School-based Student Health Survey (GSHS). Psychiatric distress was considered as the self-reported anger, anxiety, poor quality sleep, confusion, sadness/depression, worry, and violence-related behaviors (physical fight, having bully, or getting bullied).
RESULTS:
Forty percent had serum 25(OH)D values below 10 ng/mL (vitamin D deficient), and 39 % had levels 10-30 ng/mL (vitamin D insufficient). The prevalence of self-reported anger, anxiety, poor quality sleep, sadness/depression, and worry was significantly lower ($P < 0.05$) in vitamin D sufficient participants compared with their other counterparts. The odds of reporting anger, anxiety, poor quality sleep, and worry, increased approximately 1.5 to 1.8 times in

vitamin D insufficient compared with normal children and adolescents ($P < 0.05$). Risk estimates indicated that vitamin D insufficient and deficient subjects had higher odds of reporting worry compared to normal vitamin D group [OR = 2.417 (95 % CI: 1.483-3.940) for vitamin D insufficient students, and OR = 2.209 (95 % CI: 1.351-3.611) for vitamin D deficient students] (P-trend = 0.001). Violence behaviors did not show any association with vitamin D status ($P > 0.05$).

CONCLUSION:

Some psychiatric distress such as anger, anxiety, poor quality sleep, depression, and worry are associated with hypovitaminosis D in adolescents. The clinical significance of the current findings should be determined in future longitudinal studies.

KEYWORDS:

Adolescents; Anger; Anxiety; Depression; Mental health; Violence behaviors; Vitamin D

PMID: 26203431 PMCID: PMC4511535 DOI: 10.1186/s40200-015-0191-9

[PubMed] Free PMC Article

Iron and Anger

Low levels of iron can cause anger in men and women.
Low levels of iron are usually more frequent in women.

Biol Trace Elem Res. 2015 Dec;168(2):520-1. doi: 10.1007/s12011-015-0531-0.
Erratum to: Iron Deficiency Without Anemia Is Associated with Anger and Fatigue in Young Japanese Women.
Sawada T1, Konomi A2, Yokoi K3.
Author information
Erratum for
Iron deficiency without anemia is associated with anger and fatigue in young Japanese women. [Biol Trace Elem Res. 2014]
PMID: 26487444 DOI: 10.1007/s12011-015-0531-0
[PubMed]

Dairy and Anger

Diary can improve mood and lessen anger.

The Association between Dairy Intake, Simple Sugars and Body Mass Index with Expression and Extent of Anger in Female Students.

Kalantari N1, Doaei S2, Gordali M3, Rahimzadeh G4, Gholamalizadeh M5.

Author information

Abstract

OBJECTIVE:

A significant increase in violence in the world and its impact on public health and society can be an important reason to offer solutions to reduce or control anger. Studies have shown that specific food groups may be effective in controlling mental disorders such as depression, anxiety and anger. The purpose of this study was to determine the relationship between food intake and Body Mass Index on state-trait anger expression in female students of Shahid Beheshti University of Medical Sciences.

METHOD:

In this cross-sectional study, 114 female students were randomly selected from dormitories of Shahid Beheshti University of Medical Sciences. Body height and weight were measured using the scale and stadiometer, respectively. The required data for evaluating the relationship between state-trait anger expression and food consumption groups were collected using State-Trait Anger Expression Inventory-2

(STAXI-2) and Food Frequency questionnaires.

RESULTS:

The results revealed a significant negative correlation between consumption of dairy product and trait anger (angry reaction), (P = 0.015). This association remained significant after adjustment of confounding factors. No significant correlations were found between other food groups as well as BMI and state-trait anger expression.

CONCLUSION:

The higher intake of dairy products reduced state-trait anger expression. This result is consistent with the findings of many studies on the effect of dairy consumption on mental disorders. **Therefore, consumption of dairy products can be a solution for reducing anger.**

KEYWORDS:

Anger; Body Mass Index; Food Intake

PMID: 27252768 PMCID: PMC4888140

[PubMed] Free PMC Article

Leucine May Fight Anger

Take this with a grain of potassium salt.

Appl Physiol Nutr Metab. 2011 Apr;36(2):242-53. doi: 10.1139/h10-104.
Leucine-protein supplemented recovery feeding enhances subsequent cycling performance in well-trained men.
Thomson JS1, Ali A, Rowlands DS.
Author information
Abstract
The purpose of this study was to determine whether a practical leucine-protein, high-carbohydrate postexercise feeding regimen could improve recovery, as measured by subsequent cycling performance and mechanistic markers, relative to control feeding. In a crossover, 10 male cyclists performed 2- to 2.5-h interval training bouts on 3 consecutive evenings, ingesting either leucine-protein, high-carbohydrate nutrition (0.1/0.4/1.2/0.2 g·kg(-1)·h(-1); leucine, protein, carbohydrate, fat, respectively) or isocaloric control (0.06/1.6/0.2 g·kg(-1)·h(-1); protein, carbohydrate, fat, respectively) nutrition for 1.5 h postexercise. Throughout the experimental period diet was controlled, energy and macronutrient intake balanced, and protein intake clamped at 1.6 g·kg(-1)·day(-1). The alternate supplement was

provided the next morning, thereby isolating the postexercise nutrition effect. Following 39 h of recovery, cyclists performed a repeat-sprint performance test. Postexercise leucine-protein ingestion improved mean sprint power by 2.5% (99% confidence limit, ±2.6%; p = 0.013) and reduced perceived overall tiredness during the sprints by 13% (90% confidence limit, ±9.2%), but perceptions of leg tiredness and soreness were unaffected. Before exercise, creatine-kinase concentration was lowered by 19% (90% confidence limits, ±18%), but lactate dehydrogenase and pressure-pain threshold were unaltered. **There was a small reduction in anger** (25% ± 18%), but other moods were unchanged. Plasma leucine (3-fold) and essential amino acid (47%) concentrations were elevated postexercise. Net nitrogen balance trended mildly negative in both conditions (mean ± SD: leucine-protein, -20 ± 46 mg·kg(-1) per 24 h; control, -25 ± 36 mg·kg(-1) per 24 h). The ingestion of a leucine-protein supplement along with other high-carbohydrate food following intense training on consecutive days enhances subsequent high-intensity endurance performance and may attenuate muscle membrane disruption in well-trained male cyclists.
PMID: 21609286 DOI: 10.1139/h10-104
[PubMed - indexed for MEDLINE]

Controlling Anger with Medication

Medication can help with anger management. The drugs of choice depend on the cause of the anger.

Psychiatr Clin North Am. 1997 Jun;20(2):427-51.
Psychopharmacologic treatment of pathologic aggression.
Fava M1.
Author information
Abstract

Several drugs are apparently effective in treating pathologic anger and aggression. Because many of the studies on aggressive populations allowed the use of concomitant medications, it is unclear whether the efficacy of each drug in a particular population is dependent on the presence of other medications, such as antipsychotic agents. Finally, one needs to be circumspect in inferring efficacy of a particular drug in aggressive patients with neuropsychiatric conditions other than the ones in which some efficacy has been established. Lithium appears to be an effective treatment of aggression among nonepileptic prison inmates, mentally retarded and handicapped patients, and among conduct-disordered children with explosive behavior. Certainly, lithium would be the treatment of choice in bipolar patients with excessive irritability and anger outbursts, and it has been shown to be effective in this population. Anticonvulsant medications are the treatment of choice for patients with outbursts of rage and abnormal EEG findings. The efficacy of these drugs in patients without a seizure disorder, however, remains to be established, with the exception perhaps of valproate and carbamazepine. In fact, dyphenylhydantoin did not appear to be effective in treating aggressive behavior in children with temper tantrums and was found to be effective in only a prison population. There is some evidence for the efficacy of carbamazepine and valproate in treating pathologic aggression in patients with dementia, organic brain syndrome, psychosis, and personality disorders. As Yudofsky et al point out in their review of the literature, although traditional antipsychotic drugs have been used widely to treat aggression, there is little evidence for their effectiveness in treating aggression beyond their sedative effect in agitated patients or their antiaggressive effect among patients whose aggression is related to active psychosis. Antipsychotic agents appear to be effective in treating psychotic aggressive patients, conduct-disordered children, and mentally retarded patients, with only modest effects in the management of pathologic aggression in patients with dementia. Furthermore, at least in one study, these drugs were found to be associated with increased aggressiveness in mentally retarded subjects. On the other hand, atypical antipsychotic agents (i.e., clozapine, risperidone, and olanzapine) may be more effective than traditional antipsychotic drugs in aggressive and violent populations, as they have shown efficacy in patients with dementia, brain injury, mental retardation, and personality disorders. Similarly, benzodiazepines can reduce agitation and irritability in elderly and demented populations, but they also can induce behavioral disinhibition. Therefore, one should be careful in using this class of drugs in patients with pathologic aggression. Beta-blockers appear to be effective in many different neuropsychiatric conditions. These drugs seem effective in reducing violent and assaultive behavior in patients with dementia, brain injury, schizophrenia, mental retardation, and organic brain syndrome. As pointed out by Campbell et al in their review of the literature, however, systematic research is lacking, and little is known about the efficacy and safety of beta-blockers in children and adolescents with pathologic aggression. Although widely used in the management of pathologic aggression, the use of this class of drugs has been limited partially by marked hypotension and bradycardia, which are side effects common at the higher doses. The usefulness of the antihypertensive drug clonidine in the treatment of pathologic aggression has not been assessed adequately, and only marginal benefits were observed with this drug

in irritable autistic and conduct disorder children. Psychostimulants seem to be effective in reducing aggressiveness in brain-injured patients as well as in violent adolescents with oppositional or conduct disorders, particu
PMID: 9196923
[PubMed - indexed for MEDLINE]

Aspirin, Antidepressants, and Anger

According to the following article, NSAIDs or Nonsteroidal Anti-Inflammatory Drugs like aspirin can help the functioning and Cox-2 inhibitors may help SSRI antidepressant medication to work better, SSRIs are a mainstay in severe anger management.

Brain Behav. 2015 Aug;5(8):e00338. doi: 10.1002/brb3.338. Epub 2015 May 29.
Inflammation and depression: combined use of selective serotonin reuptake inhibitors and NSAIDs or paracetamol and psychiatric outcomes.
Köhler O1, Petersen L2, Mors O1, Gasse C3.

Author information
Abstract
BACKGROUND:

Nonsteroidal anti-inflammatory drugs (NSAIDs) and paracetamol have been shown to yield the potential of adjunctive antidepressant treatment effects to selective serotonin reuptake inhibitors (SSRIs); however, when investigating treatment effects of concomitant use, simultaneous evaluation of potential adverse events is important. The objective was thus to investigate treatment effectiveness and safety aspects of concomitant SSRI use with NSAIDs or paracetamol.

METHODS:

Within a 25% random sample of the Danish population, we identified all incident SSRI users between 1997 and 2006 (N = 123,351). Effectiveness and safety measures were compared between periods of SSRI use only and periods of combined SSRI and NSAID or paracetamol use by applying Cox regression.

RESULTS:

Among 123,351 SSRI users (follow-up: 53,697.8 person-years), 21,666 (17.5%) used NSAIDs and 10,232 (8.3%) paracetamol concomitantly. Concomitant NSAID use increased the risk of any psychiatric contact [Hazard rate ratio (95%-confidence interval): 1.22 (1.07; 1.38)] and with depression [1.31 (1.11;

1.55)]. Low-dose acetylsalicylic acid reduced the risk of psychiatric contact in general [0.74 (0.56; 0.98)] and with depression [0.71 (0.50; 1.01)]. Ibuprofen reduced the risk of psychiatric contacts [0.76 (0.60; 0.98)]. Concerning safety, paracetamol was associated with increased mortality [3.18 (2.83; 3.58)], especially cardiovascular [2.51 (1.93; 3.28)]. Diclofenac [1.77 (1.22; 2.55)] and the selective COX-2 inhibitors [1.75 (1.21; 2.53)] increased mortality risks.

CONCLUSIONS:

Concomitant use of SSRIs and NSAIDs occurred frequently, and effectiveness and safety outcomes varied across individual NSAIDs. Especially low-dose acetylsalicylic acid may represent an adjunctive antidepressant treatment option. The increased mortality risk of concomitant use of paracetamol needs further investigation.

KEYWORDS:

Antidepressants; depression; epidemiology; mood disorders; pharmacoepidemiology; pharmacotherapy
PMID: 26357585 PMCID: PMC4559013 DOI: 10.1002/brb3.338

Risperidone and Anger

Risperdal otherwise known as Risperidone is the most potent anger management medication of which I am am aware. At even very low doses, which cause almost no side-effects it can help even the most severe cases of anger and rage. Olanzapine, or Zyprexa, also can help with anger. Other atypical antipsychotics have demonstrated little to no ability to fight anger, indeed some may, infrequently, allow suicidal and homicidal ideation to develop.

Indian J Psychol Med. 2010 Jan;32(1):17-21. doi: 10.4103/0253-7176.70522.
An Open-label Trial of Risperidone and Fluoxetine in Children with Autistic Disorder.
Desousa A1.
Author information
Abstract
OBJECTIVE:
Various studies have shown the effectiveness of risperidone and fluoxetine in the management of behavioral problems in autism.
AIM:
The purpose of this study was to compare these two drugs in the management of behavioral problems in autism.
MATERIALS AND METHODS:

Forty children with autism were divided into 2 groups in a 16-week open trial that compared these two drugs. Parents rated the children using the Aberrant Behavior Checklist (ABC) and the Conners' Parent Rating Scale - Revised (CPRS-R). The author rated the children using the Children's Psychiatric Rating Scale and Clinical Global Impression (CGI) Scale.

RESULTS:

The risperidone group showed significant improvement in areas like irritability and hyperactivity, while the fluoxetine group showed significant improvement in speech deviance, social withdrawal and stereotypy. When the two drugs were compared, fluoxetine showed greater improvement in stereotypy, while both drugs showed improvement on the general autism scale; and on anger, hyperactivity and irritability scales.

CONCLUSIONS:

In this open trial, both drugs were well tolerated and appeared to be beneficial in the treatment of common behavioral problems in children with autism. Further controlled and double-blind studies in larger samples are warranted.

KEYWORDS:

Autistic disorder; fluoxetine; risperidone

PMID: 21799554 PMCID: PMC3137806 DOI: 10.4103/0253-7176.70522

About the author:

Will is the author of thirty popular Kindle books in English, Spanish, and French which have gone to #1 in the USA and have sold in Canada, the United Kingdom, Spain, Mexico, Argentina, France, Germany, India, Australia, Italy, and Japan. He is a former Columbia University/NYSPI Medical Library Chief, designer, and he is a speaker of English, Spanish, French, and Portuguese.

Mr. Jiang's critically-acclaimed autobiography is "A Schizophrenic Will: A Story of Madness, A Story of Hope." Mr Jiang and his intense 20+ year struggle with schizophrenia is iconoclastic because he challenges us to think differently about stereotypes of mental illness. His peers would be world movers like Philip K. Dick, John Nash, and Elyn Saks. Most movies and media news paint one-dimensional, thinly drawn caricatures of mentally ill people, instilling fear. Refreshingly, words that could describe

Mr. Jiang's life and work include: brilliant, passionate, artistic, profound, knowledgeable, inspirational, and even "wise teacher". Mr. Jiang's magnum opus in the field of psychiatry is "Guide to Natural Mental Health: Anxiety, Bipolar, Depression, Schizophrenia, and Digital Addiction: Nutrition, and Complementary Therapies" where Mr. Jiang shares deep insights into non-pharmaceutical natural strategies that are all-too-needed in this world of Big Macs and XBoxes.

William Jiang, MLS
Facebook Group: Living Well With Schizophrenia
Author Blog: http://www.mentalhealthbooks.net

Discover other titles by William Jiang, MLS

Kindle Books in English

World Traveller Social Travel Guides

Have Fun in Paris: A Guide to the Living City (Have Fun World Collection)
Have Fun in London: A Guide to the Living City (Have Fun World Collection)
Have Fun in New York A Guide to the Living City (Have Fun World Connection)
Have Fun in Rio de Janeiro: A Guide to the Living City (Have Fun World Collection)
Have Fun in Madrid: A Guide to the Living City (Have Fun World Collection)
Have Fun in Miami: A Guide to the Living City (Have Fun World Collection)
Have Fun in Boston: A Guide to the Living City (Have Fun World Collection)

About Health

A Schizophrenic Will: A Story of Madness, A Story of Hope
Guide to Natural Mental Health: Anxiety, Bipolar, Depression, Schizophrenia, and Digital Addiction: Nutrition, and Complementary Therapies, 3rd edition
Guide to Natural Intelligence Enhancement: The Medical Librarian's Annotated Guide
Natural Weight Loss and Diabetes Control: The Medical Librarian's Annotated Guide
The Medical Librarian's Guide to the Best Medicine in America

Language Guides

Tackling Spanish The Easy Way
Tackling French The Easy Way
Tackling Portuguese the Easy Way

Literature and Poetry

The Poet of Washington Heights: A Scrapbook of Poetry, Photography, Digital Art, and Social Media

Kindle Books about Ecommerce - History - Library Science

How to Shop Online like A Boss: How to do Online Consumer Shopping Right in the United States
A Historical Reader: The New York Times and Madness, 1851-1922
The English Virtual Library

Spanish

Entre la Esquizofrenia y Mi Voluntad: Una Historia de Locura y Esperanza - Jorge Alvarado, Traductor
La guía del Bibliotecario Médico: Ansiedad, Depresión, Bipolar, y Esquizofrenia: Nutrición y Terapias Complementarias, Jorge Alvarado, Traductor
Inglés Fácilmente

La Guía del Bibliotecario Médico: Sobre las Ciberadicciones

La Guía del Bibliotecario Médico: la Mejor Medicina en los Estados Unidos

Guía para Divertirse en Nueva York: Conozcan a los Neoyorquinos, Comer en los Restaurantes Mejores, Hagan Shopping Como un Jefe, Disfruten Eventos Culturales Fantásticos, y Mucho Más

French

Un Homme New Yorkais avec la Schizophrénie: Une Autobiographie

Book Teaser...

Guide to Natural Mental Health:
Anxiety, Bipolar, Depression, Schizophrenia, and Digital Addiction: Nutrition, and Complementary Therapies, 3nd Edition
By William Jiang, MLS

Foreword to the Third Edition
By William Jiang, MLS

Mental illness is still a widespread and serious problem. Currently, the the National Institute for Mental Health (NIMH) estimates about 26.2 percent of Americans ages 18 and older meet the criteria for at least one serious mental disorder, more than one in four Americans. According to another source as of 2014, the incidence of mental illness has doubled for children since the nineties. The World Health Organization (WHO) estimates that by the year 2020, depression will be the second most common cause of disability and premature death worldwide.

The statistics are grim and the problem is real and growing, but what can we do? This book tackles that very question for those who are currently suffering and those who may wish to avoid serious mental problems in the future. The good news is there is hope for many to better live with, and for some, completely avoid mental problems. The book is not meant to be seen as a panacea; rather, it offers strategies to cope with and possibly prevent mental disease that are backed up by current medical and scientific knowledge.

Although renamed, like the first edition, this book is what librarians call an annotated bibliography. This annotated bibliography picks the "best" information from the medical literature, includes commentary as well as the source, title, and abstract of the article from MEDLINE. In this case, the strength of this particular annotated bibliography is the concentration of the knowledge of world-class experts from many medical disciplines, all in one small volume, with FREE FULLTEXT for further exploration often available for more in-depth reading and learning.

This third edition includes the new topic of Digital Addiction. Complementary and alternative treatments for Digital Addiction are not included as they would most likely resemble a mixture of treatments for depression and anxiety, mostly. Digital Addiction is included to raise awareness of the relatively new and increasingly problematic constellation of electronic addictions ranging from out-of-control texting via cellular telephone to Facebook addiction to video game addiction and beyond.
To your health!

William Jiang, MLS

I was the Chief Librarian of the New York State Psychiatric Institute Patient and Family Library, affiliated with Columbia University, for seven years. This book focuses on the knowledge about Complementary and Alternative Health treatments for select mental issues that I gleaned over seven years of following the mental health literature during that time. The thrust of the book is mental health, nutrition, and complementary therapies.

Grandma Was Right

By William Jiang, MLS

Today everything is about Facebook, Twitter, and the PlayStation 3. Yet, the incidence of autism is rising, the incidence of depression is rising, the incidence of diabetes is rising, and the incidence of many other illnesses are rising. I'm not saying that grandma knew everything, but she knew what she was talking about.

Grandma said, "Go out and play!" She was so right! By going out and playing you got: one, exercise and two, sunshine. Both exercise and sunshine have been shown efficacious for treating depression once a person has it. Might it also not be a preventative? Kids these days are eating too many unhealthy foods and playing their Xbox too long. So not only do they not get exercise or Sun, they compound the problems with unhealthy foods which can cause even more problems. Childhood obesity rates are through the roof. Johnny, get off the Xbox and go play some basketball.

Grandma said, "People who live near the equator are happier." She was so right. It turns out that people in Scandinavian countries as well as other countries that don't get enough light suffer more from seasonal affective disorder which is a type of depression. However, there are many people in countries that do have enough light that also suffer from a type of seasonal affective disorder. Because they are in their offices and homes so much they don't get enough light, so the outcome is the same. There is an entire field that studies the effects of light on people's moods is called chronotherapeutics. It is a young field; but it has been shown that light has powerful antidepressant properties and in some cases is more efficacious, faster working, with a much better side effect profile than antidepressant drugs.

Grandma said, "Eat your fish; it's brain food." Boy was she right! It turns out that the Omega-3 in fish is not only good for the heart but also for the nervous system and brain. Omega-3s in fish oil has been shown to be good for mood disorders such as depression and bipolar disorder; however, less than a year ago the fish oils were shown to be efficacious in stopping schizophrenia in its tracks for people who are at high risk of developing it. Finally, fish oil also seems to have anti-inflammatory properties which can fight against the development of diabetes.

Grandma said, "Go to sleep, it's late." Grandma was right to encourage a healthy sleep schedule. It has been shown that children who go to sleep later than 10 o'clock at night are prone to more psychological problems than children who go to sleep earlier. Also, in our stressful society, it has been shown that people that get less sleep, function worse on the job. When there is a sleep deficit for many years, it can cause lasting physical problems.

Grandma said, "Eat your veggies." People do not get enough roughage these days. So, there are many people who have gastrointestinal problems that might have been prevented. Not only do the vitamins and minerals in the vegetables promote good health, the roughage is extremely important for people with bowel disorders. Eating enough fruits and vegetables decreases an unhealthy appetite so that people can lose unhealthy weight if they are overweight.

Call me a Luddite, but I think it's time to get back to basics. Don't forget to give granny a call to thank her for her wisdom.

Digital Addiction

The DSM, the Diagnostic and Statistical Manual of Mental Disorders, has been the standard for psychiatric diagnosis for the psychological and psychiatric communities since the Office of the US Surgeon General and the US Department of War published the DSM-I as a technical bulletin in 1952. The DSM was created, in large part, to help mental health workers classify shellshocked and otherwise mentally ill combat veterans who fought in World War II. The Current DSM, the DSM-V, was released at the..

Made in the USA
Monee, IL
14 October 2025